Peter

GET IN TOUCH:
WITH YOUR IDEAL WEIGHT AND OPTIMUM HEALTH

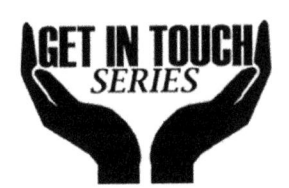

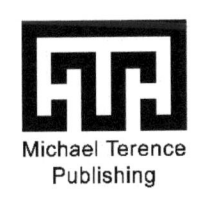

GET IN TOUCH SERIES

Michael Terence Publishing

First published in paperback by
Michael Terence Publishing in 2023
www.mtp.agency

Copyright © 2023 Peter Bull MBE

Peter Bull has asserted the right to be identified as the author of this work in accordance with the Copyright, Designs and Patents Act 1988

ISBN 9781800946750

No part of this publication may be reproduced, stored in a retrieval system, or transmitted, in any form or by any means, electronic, mechanical, photocopying, recording or otherwise, without the prior permission of the publisher

Cover images
Copyright © Peter Bull

Cover design
2023 Michael Terence Publishing

CONTENTS

PREFACE DEDICATED TO ALL FELLOW WARRIORS 1

INTRODUCTION 2

MY JOURNEY 6

INFORMATION IS NOT MOTIVATION 9

DO YOU WANT TO LOSE WEIGHT AND
    HAVE OPTIMUM HEALTH? 12

NUTRITION - WHAT NOT TO EAT 16

NUTRITION - WHAT TO EAT 19

NUTRITION - THE SECRET BENEFIT OF FASTING 22

THE FERTILISER ISSUE 25

NUTRITION - TWO TYPES OF VEGETABLE 26

NUTRITION - WHEN TO EAT 29

NUTRITION - WHERE TO EAT 31

NUTRITION - HOW TO EAT 33

NUTRITION - THE WHO OF EATING 35

PORTION SIZE AND QUANTITIES 38

NUTRITION AND WEIGHING 39

LIFESTYLE, BEHAVIOUR, OPTIMISATION 41

EXERCISE 43

PROTOCOL FOR PREVENTATIVE DIAGNOSTICS
    FOR OPTIMUM HEALTH 49

SLEEP	52
SLEEP - HOW TO GET TO SLEEP	54
BREATHING	59
RELATIONSHIPS (TURN LEFT)	62
WATER	66
SUNLIGHT	68
CONTAGIOUS DISCIPLINE	69
STRESS CONTROL	71
ABUSE	74
AVOIDING COGNITIVE DECLINE (DEMENTIA)	77
FINANCIAL SECURITY	80
GETTING CHECKED OUT	83
PATHOGENIC DISEASE	89
OPTIMUM HEALTH THROUGH A COMPLEMENTARY APPROACH	92
EMERGENCY	98
EMERGENCY - THE PRIMARY SURVEY	100
EMERGENCY - CAUSES OF UNCONSCIOUSNESS	104
ADDITIONS TO EMERGENCY PROTOCOLS	111
PRIORITISING SURVIVAL AND OPTIMUM HEALTH IN CONFLICT AND WILDERNESS SITUATIONS	115
CONCLUSION	123
FEEDBACK	124
ALSO IN THE GET IN TOUCH SERIES	125

PREFACE
Dedicated to All Fellow Warriors

All alone perched in a flat,
My friends all say You are too fat.
Come on, I hear, it's not too late
Treat yourself and lose some weight.

I'll show them those who take the rise
And scorn my gross indulgent size
Next year I'll be smart and trim
Attractive, sexy and very slim.

Fibre, calories, diets galore
Making fortunes from the weighty poor
Classes, hypnosis which do I choose
As the most effective way to lose?

The slim and lucky ones advise
All you need is exercise
Exposed by those to harassment
Uncaring of my embarrassment.

Then at last it starts to click
The weight-reducing scheme is quick
And now those jealous friends will dig
You were more-cuddly when you were big!

INTRODUCTION

Never before have health issues been more prevalent. We are living in an age of countless diets and fitness programmes, with endless advice on how to change our shape, weight and general health. Most of the planet has food issues where half the population is trying to lose weight and the other half is trying to put it on.

The problem I will be addressing in this book is that information is not motivation. I intend to prove that the more science we have on a good diet, exercise programmes and the like, the less likely we are follow the data presented. In other words, the information that is supposed to save us from ourselves is actually condemning humanity to obesity and poor health of astronomical proportions.

I will be offering a diet and lifestyle that are foolproof and cut through the endless science and research that confuses the individual to the point of inaction.

One minute, eggs are bad, the next they are good. Fats have been a sin for decades but are now encouraged in many a diet. Carbs and sugars, somewhat justifiably go through the mill of criticism, whereas protein is on the ascent. What about exercise, sleep and stress? They are all so over-researched yet there is no direct focus on well-being.

In my previous book, Get In Touch With Your Slimmer Self, I focused on the psychology of weight loss and how I managed to reduce my weight by 60 pounds in just three months. In this sequel, I am going to turn psychology into a practical approach to show you how you can lose weight effectively and keep it off. I will also describe how to obtain optimum health for your particular needs.

The benefits of this process are immense. Firstly, you will have much more energy to live an effective life. It will help you to become your real self and improve your relationships and confidence. You will lose the brain fog, fatigue and immobility associated with a poor diet. This will reduce the likelihood of many diseases, including cardiovascular, cancer, diabetes, dementia, depression and many more.

This book is not part of an extended weight loss industry with endless bolt-ons and upgrades, such as slimming classes, workout programmes, food substitutes, magazines, courses and ever-more updated further research to overwhelm the reader. It stands alone as a beacon of an enhanced lifestyle to bring contentment to anyone who follows its thinking. No one book, course or programme satisfies everyone who chooses to test out the system presented, but this book offers the majority a simple and effective way ahead. It is written for **you**, a veteran of numerous failed diets and exercise regimes. No matter how much you have failed in the past, you can now start afresh. You do not need to eat less or spend any more money on food, you simply need to change the way you think about food, health and well-being which will change the what, how, when, where and why you eat. I am confident that having read it you will never think about food, health and fitness in the same way again.

I aim to cover everything to maximise longevity and good health in one, short text. You need to go nowhere else to capture such a comprehensive guide to healthy living.

Get in Touch: With Your Ideal Weight and Optimum Health

Life offers wonderful opportunities to those who can take control of theirs. You are in control even if you don't realise it. Come with me on this journey to self-fulfilment by emailing me at

                thebestsolution@icloud.com

and let me encourage you.

Fondest regards.

Peter Bull

MY JOURNEY

Some put weight on easily; some put weight on when they eat to excess and others don't put weight on at all, no matter what they eat. I was one of those who put it on easily. At puberty, I started to get a big stomach which only grew as I got into my twenties. I was fortunate enough to have a mother who ran a slimming club so I cannot blame a lack of knowledge for not eating properly.

In my twenties, I managed to get my weight down by following the regime my mother promoted. However, I couldn't sustain it. I had quite a physical job working in the construction industry, was a keen swimmer and enjoyed squash as a ball game. I was also in the Territorial Army but despite all these incentives, I still had a large gut with plenty of flesh across my body.

Over the next thirty years, I tried everything to lose weight but having an anxious nature, I used food to comfort me when stressed. In my last book, I identified the six emotional blocks to successful weight loss: anxiety; the cold; loneliness and loss;

boredom; fatigue and socializing, where you have no control over the food that is put in front of you.

The biggest one for me was anxiety. Carbohydrates helped with my brain chemistry giving a boost to my serotonin levels which made me feel calm. The paradox was that as I felt calmer, I fretted more over my ever-increasing waistline. I felt completely out of control knowing what I should do but lacking the commitment to do it. During this period, I had a change of career and went into nursing which eventually led me to train as a psychotherapist; this helped me to understand psychology and in turn, helped my clients.

I learned that all our behaviours are a direct result of our belief system and if we have negative thinking, we will always behave in accordance with that mindset. Finally, I made a breakthrough, discovering that by changing my mindset through a certain set of techniques, I could take control without having to rely on willpower for success. This led to my writing the book Get In Touch With Your Slimmer Self.

As time passed, I gained a great deal of knowledge about diets, exercise, obesity, lifestyle, longevity and well-being to which this book is dedicated. I have developed a good diet that works for most people and in combination with exercise and the correct psychology, most overweight people across the world can achieve an optimum Body Mass Index (BMI) size and ideal weight.

I used to believe that when I stopped worrying, I would lose weight. In reality, it is the reverse. When we lose weight and have a healthy diet our anxiety reduces and I believe the other emotional enemies of weight loss will respond to losing the weight. Now I am the ideal weight and find it easy to control it.

Life is very difficult today for most of us with financial, family, health, time and work worries. We can put off the risks of obesity caused by a complex, difficult life. However, I feel this book will give you the simplest and most straight forward way to take control of your body and reduce life's difficulties in the process.

INFORMATION IS NOT MOTIVATION

For most of human existence, around one million years, people struggled to survive. They ate what they could get, initially using instinct to select the correct foods. In recent times, science, medicine and technology have made it possible for large parts of the world to survive through intensive farming and artificial fertilisers.

In the last 100 years, research has isolated fundamental food types and much study has gone into their nutritional benefits or otherwise in our diet. The problem is, as more and more research is done, society is becoming confused and demotivated. We no longer know who to believe. As knowledge increases, so does obesity. The human brain cannot cope with the dictates of an ever-changing scientific community; the result is we rebel and head for all the foods that are both fattening and lacking in optimum nutritional value.

This book will cut through all the scientific research to show you a simple programme that is based on a foolproof system that works for the vast majority of the population. It is essential that if you wish to lose weight, **you must not focus on weight but on nutrition.** It is easy to lose weight if you starve but that will eventually kill you. The paradox with all weight reduction programmes is that to get thin, you need to think about food much more than normal. A constant focus on food can lead to eating more than if you have never bothered in the first place. Too much information exacerbates this condition. We worry more about our appearance than we do about our health and it is only when our health breaks down that we start to focus on that, rather than the big stomach.

From today I would like you to treat weight loss as a health issue rather than an appearance one as this will help you to become motivated. The process is very simple. I will take each question and explain it in an easy-to-understand way. We will look at what to eat, when to eat, how to eat, where to eat, why to eat and who is doing the eating. By the end of each chapter, you should try one thing a week and slowly build up new eating habits over several weeks which will slowly change your relationship with food forever. Sudden surges in motivation where you try everything at once rarely work and are overwhelming. The brain sets down new pathways of thinking, a bit at a time. Using this method, you will change permanently. We will also look at the other factors for optimum health such as sleep, exercise and stress, using the same model of who, what, when, where, how and why.

DO YOU WANT TO LOSE WEIGHT AND HAVE OPTIMUM HEALTH?

In this chapter, I want to identify the whole issue of motivation to follow a weight-reducing, healthy diet and lifestyle in our own time.

The primary problem with the desire to lose weight is an inbuilt mindset that is temporary. People lose weight for a specific event like a wedding or for a limited time so they will look good in a bathing costume on holiday. They have already decided subconsciously that they will go back to their old ways of eating as soon as possible. People are sprinters rather than long-distance runners when it comes to motivation.

The second problem is that of instant gratification. The pleasure of food on the tongue now overrides the delayed gratification of weight loss in the future. This is mainly caused by focusing on the waistline rather than nutrition. People will not appreciate the problems of a poor diet at the time of eating. It is only when they get sick that they start to think about their general health.

How do we as an obese society deal with this problem? One solution which is a hot topic these days is using medication as an appetite suppressant. The most effective is probably Wegovy which mimics the gut hormone, GLP1. This slows down the movement of food through the gut making you stay full for longer. For some this will be a life-saver; for most, it is a temporary fix as appetite suppressants could have long-term side effects. They don't provide optimum health as your diet might be as bad as before, compromising general health. It might also stop people from converting to nutritious food as an alternative to junk food. I am sure many will benefit from a medicated intervention but quality of life needs to be holistic rather than a quick-fix solution. **The motivator is to eat more healthy food rather than to eat less rubbish food.**

Achieving all this requires a clear, focused mind. In life, we hold certain things dear, our loved ones, our families, our work and our passions. Sadly, for many obese people, losing weight is not the priority they think it is. If you seriously want to lose weight it has to be the most important activity in your life. To attempt to lose it half-heartedly will end in failure. We don't need more education, we need more action.

All activities worth doing require effort. The effort of selecting the correct foods. The effort of cooking in some incidences. The effort of shaping our day to correspond to an effective programme and so on. We need to simplify the process so there is less to demotivate us and push us off track. We also need the patience to make little changes and gradually increase them as our motivation is rewarded by small gains. You will have the complete optimum programme of what to do, when to do it, how to do it, where to do it and why to do it on the following pages.

I have mentioned here and in my previous book the six emotional barriers to weight loss. These are boredom, anxiety, fatigue, loneliness and loss, socialising and the cold. Building your motivation requires addressing some of these issues in life.

This is not only about changing your emotional state to change your eating habits, it is about changing your eating habits to change your

emotional state. Motivation comes from working on these two ideas concurrently rather than consecutively.

NUTRITION
- WHAT NOT TO EAT

There are two considerations when looking into your diet for ideal weight and optimum health. The first is general advice which is covered by the internet and the second is specific advice directed at an individual. General advice is about experts making a name and promoting their specific agenda to promote their latest book, course or presentation. This advice might be good but it does not take account of the fact that we are all different. One size does not fit all in every sense of the word.

Specific advice is designed to focus on the individual and will take into account their metabolism, genetics, lifestyle etc. In this book, I am going to attempt the impossible by giving general advice which will be specific to you as a reader of this work.

General advice tells you what you shouldn't eat and what you should eat. This book is different. I will tell you what you shouldn't eat and then you can and should eat everything else. The more variety the better but the quantities should be smaller. Obviously, there are foods that you simply hate and those you can tolerate. The healthy foods that you can tolerate are a good starting point to change, if the foods you like are of low nutritional value.

Firstly, you will need to confirm foods that are specifically bad for you as an individual. These are split into three types: foods that you are intolerant of; foods that you are allergic to and foods that you are anaphylactic to.

Food intolerance is when you can eat a food but as you eat more of it, you develop an adverse physical reaction. Skin conditions, asthma, migraine, weight gain and Irritable Bowel Syndrome (IBS) are all possible results of food intolerance.

Food allergy is where you get a reaction from very little exposure and medical issues come on quickly but are not life-threatening.

Food anaphylaxis is where you cannot tolerate any amount of the substance within a certain food group and can be life-threatening. This exposure would require immediate action giving the casualty adrenaline from an EpiPen injection. Further medical intervention at a hospital would also be required. To perform this, I recommend you look at the chapter on emergency and get some training on a recognised First Aid course.

You should consult a physician or a nutritionist and have a blood test to confirm these. Once you have established foods that you can personally take, then we need to look at foods that put weight on and are unhealthy. These are processed foods with multi-ingredients. **Single-ingredient foods are foods that come straight from nature and have not been processed, mixed by others or compounded into recipes.** Examples of single-ingredient foods are fruit, vegetables, unprocessed meat and fish.

NUTRITION - WHAT TO EAT

Once you have eradicated the foods that you should avoid, you now need to look at the good foods. These are any foods that come directly from nature and haven't been interfered with by mankind. They are all defined as single ingredients like fruit, vegetables, unprocessed meat and fish as mentioned in the last paragraph. The point is that you must eat a wider range of these foods. Five vegetables a day is no good, especially if you are eating the same five every day. You need to eat eight or more but in smaller quantities. When considering what to eat, ask yourself, has the food got an ingredient label? If so, avoid it. It will likely be processed.

Supplements

We are constantly told that our diet does not contain all the correct foodstuffs we need for a healthy life. Hence the growth and popularity of health food shops. We are also warned that supplements are not an alternative to a balanced diet. What should we believe?

The answer is very straight forward. Some people do not absorb all the nutrients naturally existing in foods. If you focus on the multi-single-ingredient programme I have already mentioned, you will be exposed to all the vitamins, electrolytes, minerals etc. necessary for a healthy life.

The inability to absorb certain primary foodstuffs can be checked with blood tests conducted by a physician or nutritionist. Some people will only discover they are lacking in something when they develop symptoms and this should be picked up when diagnosis occurs. Supplements will then be prescribed.

The other issue is that certain supplements can be overdosed and should be taken with care. The main thing is to learn about yourself and what supplements will complement your diet if necessary. Most health food shops have well-trained staff who can warn you about any risk of overdosing. Most vitamin or multivitamin tablets are ok, but always read the labels and see where the supplement could affect your health in another way. Never go over the dose stated on the label and periodically review what you are putting into your mouth. The same foodstuffs do not always have the same health benefits throughout life.

You should avoid researching every theory produced by the latest expert with a book and YouTube videos and focus on what works for you as an individual.

NUTRITION
- THE SECRET BENEFIT OF FASTING

During the past few years, there has been a massive interest in fasting as a weight loss and health intervention. There is much research both online and offline about the benefits of fasting for your physical and mental well-being.

I don't intend to go through all of that as you can get all the data you want - and more! - from the internet. My aim is to provide a little-known benefit that I believe outweighs all the others. Fasting is the quickest way to reprogramme your mind around food.

We all have cravings and unless you are pregnant, they are normally around carbohydrates, sugars and fats found predominantly in processed, multi-ingredient foods like ready-meals and take-aways. This is the result of an evolutionary process to build weight during famine and drought.

I am sure you would agree that if we could only crave nutritious, single-ingredient foods like vegetables and protein-rich foodstuffs, our problems would be over. The good news is that we can learn to crave these foods rather than the carbs, sugars etc.

This is achieved by fasting. Start by preparing some extremely healthy food like a multi-vegetable soup. It only takes minutes to prepare especially with a blender. You can add protein in the form of meat or fish unless you are a vegetarian or vegan. Either way, add spices like turmeric and ginger to give it a' kick'. When it is ready, go on a 24-hour hour fast where you eat nothing and only drink water. Check with your physician or nutritionist before you fast, as it can be unhealthy for some. When you break your fast, preferably in the morning, take a couple of bowls of soup before you eat anything else.

When you fast you become genuinely hungry and experience what many in affluent Western culture have never experienced. The brain confuses craving with real hunger. In other words, by doing this on a few occasions you will start to crave these healthy foods. I now love these nutritious foods and can't wait to have more. It might not work the first time you fast but you should try it once a week until you have reprogrammed your brain to crave healthy foods regularly.

With many healthy eating programmes, we do not get hungry enough to make this mental switch and this is worsened by the complexity of diet regimes that make us continuously think about food when trying to follow a slimming programme. The same willpower that drives us to want to forget about food pushes us to crave it more as we are always thinking about it. I have made a commitment to keep you away from too much information and fasting does just that. I do not believe fasting is for everyone and it does have to be practised with caution. However, for otherwise healthy people fasting from time to time reboots the brain into craving the 'superfoods'.

THE FERTILISER ISSUE

One issue that is difficult to manage when trying to eat a healthy diet is that of artificial fertilisers which can contaminate food before it leaves the farm. The only solution is to grow your own. This achieves several aims of this book in one activity, i.e. it is an interest, exercise, it takes place outdoors and provides fertilizer-free food.

Obviously, it is much easier if you have a garden but consider putting your name down for an allotment where you can rent land at a reasonable price to grow vegetables. Hens can also produce eggs but this is more difficult to manage in built-up areas.

There are many videos on the net as well as courses and books on how to grow vegetables, even with small amounts of land. One point to remember, you will have to dedicate some hours each week to keeping the vegetable patch up to scratch, especially with watering.

NUTRITION
- TWO TYPES OF VEGETABLE

**Salad vegetables
versus root and green vegetables**

I would like to offer you a very simple description of the vegetables you should eat for optimum health and sustained weight loss. There are essentially two types of vegetable food groups, those that can be eaten raw and those that you need to cook.

In essence, salad vegetables can be eaten raw and cold, whereas most green and root vegetables need cooking and are eaten hot. All you need to do is split your vegetable diet in two. Half of all you eat is salad vegetables and the other half is the greens and root type.

Some vegetables are transition vegetables, like tomatoes which are strictly a fruit, and carrots which can be eaten raw or cooked. That aside, you should introduce as many as you can. The cooked vegetables can all be turned into a multi-vegetable soup with small quantities of each vegetable to counteract the number you are eating. This has the benefit that the goodness which boils off into the water is also drunk, so you lose nothing. A pressure cooker or microwave is best but a saucepan with a lid will suffice. It is preferable to focus more on cooked vegetables in cold climates and raw vegetables in warmer or hot climates.

Fortunately, in Western supermarkets, the salad vegetables are separated from the root and green vegetables. It is also a good idea to split your consumption of cooked roots and greens in two. The best of all options is to eat one-third of raw salad vegetables, one-third of cooked root vegetables and one-third of cooked green vegetables.

There are many sources of protein and again the secret is to vary your protein choices as much as possible. Meat and fish should be alternated with dairy and eggs as options. Any protein foods are good, as long as the quantities are small and the variety is wide.

Modern thinking suggests it is the sugars and carbohydrates that are bad. This is true, but rather than focusing on eating less of these, focus on gives your body more time to actively work off the calories before the next sleep. Do not eat just because others are eating at a certain time. My friends are used to me having a cup of coffee when we are out for a meal if the food presented is not healthy or slimming.

Eat when you are hungry. You don't need to have food just because it is mealtime for everyone else. You can also miss a part of the meal or even eat it later. This system breaks your body's familiarity with eating habits which in turn helps weight loss.

Finally, I recommend that you always leave a bit on your plate. It might sound wasteful but it is a brilliant psychological trick to convince your subconscious that you are full. Next time, take a little bit less and leave a bit at the end. This will reduce your portion size bit by bit. Incremental changes over time can completely change your life without you even noticing it and act as one of the strongest motivators there are.

counteract the number you are eating. This has the benefit that the goodness which boils off into the water is also drunk, so you lose nothing. A pressure cooker or microwave is best but a saucepan with a lid will suffice. It is preferable to focus more on cooked vegetables in cold climates and raw vegetables in warmer or hot climates.

Fortunately, in Western supermarkets, the salad vegetables are separated from the root and green vegetables. It is also a good idea to split your consumption of cooked roots and greens in two. The best of all options is to eat one-third of raw salad vegetables, one-third of cooked root vegetables and one-third of cooked green vegetables.

There are many sources of protein and again the secret is to vary your protein choices as much as possible. Meat and fish should be alternated with dairy and eggs as options. Any protein foods are good, as long as the quantities are small and the variety is wide.

Modern thinking suggests it is the sugars and carbohydrates that are bad. This is true, but rather than focusing on eating less of these, focus on eating more of the nutritious foods. I say this because carbohydrates are found in vegetables and sugar is found in fruit. If you cut out all carbs and sugars there is little left to eat. Carbs and sugars are most damaging when found in processed food. Protein is an excellent foodstuff for making you feel full. If you are a vegan, the diet presented here will give you lots of protein as the amino acids in a wide range of vegetables will counteract the lack of meat, dairy and fish in your diet.

NUTRITION
- WHEN TO EAT

There are two things to consider about when you should eat from the weight point of view. The most important factor is the total amount of food you consume in twenty-four hours. This is the base of traditional calorie-counting. The theory goes, the fewer calories you put in, the less weight you will put on. This is only a partial answer as the time of day you eat will affect your digestive system and the levels of motivation to avoid overeating. I believe in the delay principle which I call the 'Micro fast'. This states that once you have analysed your daily eating patterns, try delaying a certain food indulgence for an extra two minutes each day. If you eat just before bedtime, say at 11 pm, then stop eating at 10.58 pm the following day. On day three, stop eating at 10.56 pm and so on. Two minutes is nothing but when compounded over some weeks, this will desensitise your craving to eat.

It is best to eat the bulk of your food early in the day or after sleep if you are working night shifts. This gives your body more time to actively work off the calories before the next sleep. Do not eat just because others are eating at a certain time. My friends are used to me having a cup of coffee when we are out for a meal if the food presented is not healthy or slimming.

Eat when you are hungry. You don't need to have food just because it is mealtime for everyone else. You can also miss a part of the meal or even eat it later. This system breaks your body's familiarity with eating habits which in turn helps weight loss.

Finally, I recommend that you always leave a bit on your plate. It might sound wasteful but it is a brilliant psychological trick to convince your subconscious that you are full. Next time, take a little bit less and leave a bit at the end. This will reduce your portion size bit by bit. Incremental changes over time can completely change your life without you even noticing it and act as one of the strongest motivators there are.

NUTRITION
- WHERE TO EAT

Some places are conducive to weight loss and some are not. The more control you have over the food facing you, the more weight you will lose. Reduce the times you eat out or ensure that where you eat has single-ingredient foods where you can help yourself. The best examples are salad bars, healthy buffets and some diners.

When you find these, you can eat larger quantities of multiple, single-ingredient fruit and vegetables which will improve your weight situation massively.

If this is not possible, start on the super soup. This takes only a few minutes to make and will contain as many blended vegetables as you can get in a saucepan. Each time you make it, try to add another vegetable and cut down on the amount of each vegetable in a direct ratio to the one you are introducing. I have managed to include eight vegetables and spices so far and am aiming for 12 in the next few months.

Many supermarkets don't provide a wide range of vegetables, so you will have to hunt far and away to find more.

It is rather like taking a multivitamin, a small pill with many different vitamins in tiny quantities.

Plan where you will eat your meals, preferably at a table, and ritualise the experience. The ideal is to eat as a family taking as long as possible to finish your meal. Eating on your lap in front of the TV is tantamount to weight gain.

NUTRITION
- HOW TO EAT

Is there a way to eat that will actually help you lose weight? I believe there is and the following chapter will show you how. It takes around 20 minutes for the brain to register that you have eaten and this delay is where most of the weight is put on. You don't know you are satisfied for twenty minutes so you go on eating during that period.

The secret to solving this problem is to eat much more slowly. The slower you eat, the more weight you will lose. There are three ways to slow down your eating. Firstly, never eat if you are in a hurry. Save your food until you have an opportunity to take it slowly. Secondly, you should count to ten in your head between mouthfuls. Over time, you should increase this number to fifteen and twenty etc. The third way to slow down your eating is to chew your food for longer before you swallow it. If you are eating something like soup that you cannot chew you will need to pretend to chew the food by moving your jaw ten to twenty times before taking the next mouthful. Over time, your eating will slow down to a point where satisfaction will kick in. By the end of the meal, this will have reduced the desire to eat to excess. The whole thing might sound crazy, but it works. It also has the added benefit of improving your digestion, reducing symptoms of IBS and acid reflux.

NUTRITION
- THE WHO OF EATING

This chapter is all about who you associate with to secure the maximum motivation for permanent weight loss. The first association is a slimming group. These can be both very good and very bad. We get a great deal of motivation by associating with fellow travellers in the world of weight reduction, people who understand what we are going through and when we see an associate losing weight, it gives us hope.

Unfortunately, there is a demotivating side to slimming groups and that is their programme model. Today, slimming groups are mainly commercial concerns generating billions of dollars across the globe to help people lose weight. There is a built-in inertia. They need you to remain a member for a long time to secure their continuous funding. If you lose well and stop coming back for weekly or online meetings, it undermines their financial base.

To achieve this commitment, they will throw masses of food technology at you with various counting schemes to keep you on track. It becomes a pseudo-science with invented formulas created by the group that are very confusing. The obsession is transferred from losing weight to following the ever-more complex dieting programme. Individuals get caught up in the trivia of the system, spending the meeting discussing their weekly intake. This is a petty approach which locks the obese into a yoyo round of fighting weight, lasting a lifetime. They never really crack the issue because their motivation is prevented from thriving by trivial detail.

The second 'Who' of weight loss motivation is the spiritual support group. These groups do not deal with the programme but focus on the emotional elements of overeating which include boredom, loneliness and loss, anxiety, depression, cold temperatures, socialising and fatigue. The basis of this method is to heal the emotional wounds and the weight will come off on its own. They are good but have to be translated into a simple replacement diet that does not reinforce the emotional effect. Having mentors, sponsors, relatives and friends can also help but if they are too close, resentment and personality clashes will interfere with progress. I do not disparage any of the above and if it works for you, keep doing whatever is working. All I say is select your counsel carefully and remember some will offer all sorts of remedies at a price.

PORTION SIZE AND QUANTITIES

In this book, I am suggesting a different way of thinking. Almost all the existing programmes for weight loss are formulaic, where the expert tells you what to eat to lose weight. As I am sure you will agree, this is not working as obesity is getting worse. I have deliberately avoided telling you how much to eat as this data is highly demotivating. Weight loss is not a formula, it is an attitude of mind. You will soon discover exactly how much you need to eat to keep losing weight. Your goal is to stop focusing on amounts and focus on variety.

A portion is the amount of any food that you can fit into your hand. If that is a single-ingredient food, you can eat it. However, as you progress you can split that food into two single-ingredient foods with the same portion size within your hand. You should focus on quality not quantity. The greater the variety in one portion the better.

NUTRITION AND WEIGHING

In my last book, I mentioned the benefits of weighing your food rather than yourself. I would like to expand on this idea in the following chapter to show how it changes mindsets.

When you are weighing yourself, you are using a way of measuring your progress for motivational purposes. If you lose weight, you assume that will make you more motivated. The problem is that when someone loses weight, they often reward themselves with the wrong kind of food. If they put on weight, they commiserate by doing the same thing. The only time weighing can have a positive effect is if the weight stays the same.

However, weighers become weighing junkies, starting to play games with themselves, like changing the time of day to weigh, weighing before using the toilet then after their next visit to the bathroom. Another self-deception is the change of clothing each time we weigh. All of these are a form of denial to get the scales to lie in our favour. I recommend you weigh yourself at most once a week and preferably longer. Once a month is probably the optimum amount of time between weigh-ins.

Alternatively, you can start weighing your food. It doesn't matter how much it weighs as you will be able to reduce it in tiny amounts over time. What matters is that you weigh it. This shifts your mind from the weight-losing mentality to the nutritional thinking. Weighing food is not emotional whereas weighing ourselves is. We cannot fight emotion with willpower so it is better to apply our will to food weighing and avoid the emotional weighing link altogether.

LIFESTYLE, BEHAVIOUR, OPTIMISATION

Optimum health requires optimisation. Many people are working from home these days and as such can adjust their time better. However, the problem is that the discipline of attending work helped them structure their day. This day was controlled by others who directed individual behaviour. However, when they got home they were too tired to think about preparing food and exercising. Sleep is something they neglected as they wanted to reward themselves for their hard work and would stay up late, overeating too close to bedtime and failing to exercise. They had used up their motivational store at work and couldn't be bothered to delay their gratification to get healthy. How much nicer to indulge and get that dopamine fix associated with so many unhealthy activities!

Those who work from home are in a much stronger position to improve their health by their own efforts. They can often dovetail their work around their healthy living habits rather than sandwiching their health around their work. This slight change of emphasis will not only help their general fitness but will incidentally help their work performance as well. Heathy, fit people work better than those who aren't.

EXERCISE

It is universally agreed by all the experts that exercise is beneficial to humanity as a whole. Exercise plays many roles in optimum health and within certain limits, the more you do the better.

For many adults, returning to exercise since childhood, their initial motivation is to lose weight. I would like to use equivocation to define the power of exercise as a weight-losing feature. Exercise helps you lose weight and not lose weight at the same time. The effects of how much exercise you need to do to work off the calories of just one biscuit would leave you permanently in the gym. The vast majority of weight loss is concerned with what you put in your mouth. Some have found that exercise can turn fat into muscle and weight is gained. How then can exercise help you to lose weight?

Exercise will motivate you to consistently change your bad eating habits. This has a much greater effect than just burning calories and is much more associated with self-discipline. People see weight loss through healthy eating as an activity of denial, whereas exercise is an active pursuit. When exercising, you are producing chemicals in the body such as endorphins that give you a chemical 'high'. This high can become addictive. There is a very small step from this addiction to an addiction to nutritious foods. On days when you are not exercising, follow the intermittent fasting programme mentioned earlier and mentally anchor this rush to eating nutritious food. Food science tells us when, how, where and what to eat and is factual. It lacks emotional input, but exercise has this emotional element through endorphin release.

There is so much data regarding exercise that it is impossible to keep up, so I have decided to summarise it in the following points.

1 Amount of exercise

Any exercise is better than none, provided you don't go beyond your health tolerance limit. Consult a physician or personal trainer for advice on this, the more the merrier.

2 Types of exercise

a) Aerobic (cardiovascular) - anaerobic (weight training).

You should do a mix of both, working up slowly. Weights are best done in a public gym to avoid injury and under the supervision of a qualified member of staff.

b) Group exercise versus individual exercise.

Are you more motivated in groups like aerobic or circuit classes or do you prefer to work on your own?

c) Competitive exercise versus non-competitive.

A further subdivision of group exercise is sport where a group is usually chasing a ball. This form of teamwork works well for those who love to compete but don't want to exercise for its own sake.

d) Social exercise

This is the hidden form that responds to the power of rhythmic music and is called dancing. Never underestimate the incredible amount of physical exertion gained from going to clubs, raves and discos. This is mainly for the younger population who need exercise more today than ever before.

Note: take ear protectors with you as hearing loss can increase over time.

3 When to exercise

Whenever you get a chance. The cheapest and most effective form of long-term exercise for health is walking. The more you walk, the fitter you get. Mankind is designed to walk. He is not designed to run marathons or kick a ball about, but walking is universal for all able-bodied people. 10,000 steps a day can be easily achieved if you walk locally during an active day rather than taking mechanical transport.

4 Where to exercise

The best place to exercise is outdoors, provided the air quality is acceptable and you don't suffer from serious respiratory conditions. Those seasonally affected by pollen are probably better exercising in towns, but for all others the countryside is ideal. Plants and especially trees will absorb much of a region's pollution and provide fresh oxygen for good respiration.

5 How to exercise

A secret of optimum health can be described as 'everything in moderation'. The real reason is more like 'variety is the spice of life'. The more varied your exercise routine, the fitter you become. However, progressive exercise has the best long-lasting results. Progressive exercise follows the FITT principle and you never do exactly the same thing twice.

FITT stands for Frequency, Intensity, Time, and Type. Each time you exercise, change one feature. With Frequency, you might increase your visits to the gym or do a second set of reps on weights. Intensity works on how hard the programme is within a fixed time. Four kilometres in thirty minutes on one day will be set at four-and-a-half in half an hour on the next visit.

Time is largely to do with endurance and involves the length of time you are exercising. A thirty-minute workout on one occasion becomes a thirty-five-minute workout on the subsequent occasion.

Type is, as mentioned above, one time you focus on weights, another time cardio, the next, going for a cross-country run, the next a game of basketball followed by a swim. The more varied, the fitter you become. The body soon gets used to a certain exercise and the benefit will diminish in time.

Finally, when doing progressive exercise, only change one thing at a time. Do not go from running one mile in fifteen minutes to running two miles in ten minutes. The smaller the change and the more often that change occurs, the more you will experience long-term improvements.

PROTOCOL FOR PREVENTATIVE DIAGNOSTICS FOR OPTIMUM HEALTH

To establish optimum health, we need to assume that we start with good health as default and our behaviour causes it to break down. Of course, genetics do not guarantee good health for everyone but other factors are negotiable.

The protocol is broken up into seven elements: Definition; Causes; Signs; Symptoms; Prognosis; History and Treatment/avoiding procedures. To help keep it simple, here's an example.

Definition

High blood pressure (Hypertension)

Firstly, it is important to understand that hypertension consists of two raised readings, the systolic and the diastolic. The definition of hypertension is therefore a blood pressure where one or both of these readings is above a recommended level. In older people, it would be around 140/90 as a cutoff.

When these readings are elevated, that suggests high blood pressure.

Causes

The causes vary, including, temporary versus long-term high blood pressure, being overweight, being stressed, a poor diet, familial and genetic factors, and lack of aerobic exercise.

Signs, symptoms, history and prognosis

The signs, i.e. what a health care professional sees, and symptoms, i.e. what the individual tells the professional during a consultation, are often hidden with blood pressure. If you are suffering from shock, you will experience an ashen-grey face, high heart rate and rapid shallow breathing. Blood pressure, on the other hand, would need checking with a machine to confirm the diagnosis. These signs and symptoms would be backed up by a history of hypertension in the family or from previous visits to a physician by the patient. Finally, a prognosis is made as to what might happen if the condition is not addressed. Stress-related Blood Pressure might simply be due to having it taken. This is known as 'white coat syndrome, a fear of medical checks.

Treatment

Once diagnostics have confirmed the high blood pressure, a regime is recommended to reduce it. This would include medication, weight loss, exercise, blood pressure-reducing foods and stress management. The secret of effective treatment is to do as many of these as appropriate to ensure a long-term result. With 'white coat syndrome', regular checks or checking at home with your own machine would normalise the results.

These protocols can be applied to any condition that might threaten optimum health at any time in life. So, to restate them, remember:

1 Definition - (What is it?)

2 Causes - (How do you get it?)

3 Signs - (What someone sees or tests for it)

4 Symptoms - (What a patient describes about it)

5 History - (What long-term behaviour led up to it?)

6 Potential prognosis - (What happens if not treated?)

7 Treatment - (How do you treat it?)

SLEEP

The way we have been designed requires us to spend a third of our lives in an unconscious state of sleep. It is a vital component of optimum health and is as important as exercise and diet.

Why we need sleep

More repair of both physical and mental health problems is achieved during sleep than during our waking hours. We do not consciously work on this repair, it is automatic. We do, however, need to get enough and that is the main topic of this chapter.

I think that most interventions applied during the day to maintain and improve our well-being and general health are a preparation for the sleep experience. Please do not ignore this very important part of life as it changes everything. Did you notice that if you have enough sleep, it will motivate you to change your diet and exercise? It will also consolidate the knowledge to obtain optimum health permanently.

The first element of sleep to be considered is how much you are getting. The second is the quality of sleep and the third is how to get optimum sleep if you suffer from insomnia.

SLEEP
- HOW TO GET TO SLEEP

This book is designed to be straightforward forward so I am not going to go into the whole science of sleep. If you have trouble sleeping, you need to rule out a physical cause of insomnia. This might be pain, sickness or stress keeping you awake. This requires medical intervention.

However, there are other causes of poor sleep and one needs a mention. When someone goes to bed and seems to sleep for many hours but still feels tired, they might be suffering from sleep apnea. This condition is often associated with snoring but snoring is not always relevant. Sleep apnea causes short spurts of stopping breathing which triggers the individual to wake up multiple times during the night. Once diagnosed, there are ways of improving the effects by using a breathing machine to allow air to flow. You can also consider issues like postnasal drip and sleeping on your back. Ensure you have sufficient vitamin D and magnesium in your diet. I would recommend a multivitamin supplement but check with your pharmacist on this issue as overdose is a risk. There are hundreds of thousands if not millions of people world-wide suffering from this condition, so go to your doctor and get it checked out.

Other less acute reasons for sleep deprivation are easier to control. The first is the time you choose to retire. If you need to get up at 6 am and require 7 hours, a minimum for most people, then you will need to be in bed by 10.30 pm to approach the seven hours slot.

Eating late will also reduce your chances of getting to sleep. Digestion of food requires a great deal of energy which can keep you awake much of the night. It is recommended that you don't eat for about three hours before you go to bed. On the other hand, if you practise having a siesta, a sleep after lunch, which is popular in hot countries, having a meal can actually aid sleep. This is only useful with short spells of sleep during the day.

Make your room as dark as possible as any form of light can keep you from sleeping. If you have children who are scared of the dark, you might have to leave a light on but that aside, the darker the better.

The ideal temperature for sleep involves the body going from cold to warm when tucked under the blankets. A cold shower or even sticking your head in cold water for a few seconds can induce sleep. You won't sleep if you are too cold and you won't sleep if you are too hot but going from cold to warm will induce sleep.

Reading is a good method of inducing sleep, providing it is inane, eg a novel or fantasy. Reading work reports or studying is probably not good as it stimulates the brain and can trigger anxiety which will stop you from sleeping.

Avoid stimulating drinks like coffee but hot milk can help. Try not to drink too much before bed as even water will cause you to get up in the night to visit the toilet and disrupt your sleep pattern. If sleep is a major problem, then your doctor might recommend sleeping pills which should only be taken under supervision and are not a long-term solution. However, pain killers might help if your insomnia is due to pain.

Try to resolve any arguments or confrontations with family members before you turn in as these will play on your mind. It is also important to ensure you are comfortable with the right amount of pillow support under your head and neck to feel relaxed. If you have acid reflux, it is good to raise the top of your bed slightly - a couple of house bricks are good - so gravity keeps the stomach acid away from your oesophagus. Older people with hiatus hernias are particularly susceptible to this condition.

Mindfulness can also help you to get to sleep. This was the source of the old idea of counting sheep. I used to imagine playing squash, just hitting the ball against the wall again and again. Repetitive thoughts in the present are very effective for sleep.

If you wake up in the night and can't get to sleep, have an unpleasant job lined up like clearing a cupboard or washing the floor. The more boring the better. The twin advantages are that bed becomes an attractive option and you tick off a job you have been avoiding during the day. This idea of trying to stay awake was developed by the famous psychologist, Victor Frankl, a holocaust survivor who created the term Paradoxical Intention.

It is never a good idea to smoke but this is especially important in bed because of the risk of being burnt or a full-scale fire. People wrongly believe that smoking helps them relax but it is the deep-breathing that smokers practise when smoking that is relaxing, not the cigarette itself.

BREATHING

It is often said that if you can control your breathing, you can control your life. Working on the best breathing techniques is very powerful for getting your 'fight, flight or freeze' responses into proportion. This has the side-effect of balancing hormones that ultimately can be detrimental to health if left unchecked.

Good breathing is at the centre of many old as well as modern well-being disciplines, including Yoga, meditation and general fitness. Effective breathing has to be worked on so it becomes a habit but it is a very easy habit to master. Volumes have been written on the subject but in deference to this book, I will focus on a simple technique that works very well in most cases.

The most important consideration is to practise many times during the day. This will help break down the geographical and timed anchors that trigger negative thoughts and feelings. Correct breathing is as important as diet, exercise and sleep to provide optimum health.

Firstly, you need to be comfortable, not overly anxious, exhausted or in pain to practise this technique. This is designed as a preventative measure rather than first aid when things have got out of control.

Find a place to sit or lie down and try to avoid loud noises and all forms of distraction. Take a deep breath in and count in your head to four. When you have filled your lungs as much as possible, hold your breath for a further count of four. Finally, breathe out slowly for the count of six, seven or eight before taking the next breath. Work on breathing from the abdomen; as you breathe in, your abdomen should extend upwards. This can be measured by placing your hand on your lower chest, and as you exhale, your abdomen will retract downwards. It is also much better if you breathe in through your nose and out through your mouth.

Repeat the procedure up to ten times with each cycle lasting about 15 seconds. This equates to about four inhalations per minute. The benefits are enormous; you will feel relaxed and calm as well as energised and full of life. It will clear your head and improve your chances of success in all aspects of life. As I said, this is preventative and it is no good only doing it when stressed. The more you do it, the more you will benefit from its effects.

RELATIONSHIPS (TURN LEFT)

Modern research keeps coming up with the same conclusions. To live a long life, and have optimum health and happiness, we need meaningful close relationships. Humans, as with many of our animal cohabiters, function best within relationships.

The ideal multilevel connection is with parent, child and sibling being most important. Sexual romantic relationships are also essential for most, as life-long companionship is closely linked to contentment.

Friends come a very close second to these types of connection and will often substitute the above if individuals lack the closeness of the intimate family unit.

Groups can also act as a surrogate, especially where people live in a group setting as with institutions like the military or other close-knit occupations. We are all individuals and different relationships work differently for each person.

The essential element of any relationship is codependence; that is a commitment to the other and for them to be committed to us. This book is not just a treatise in social study, it is written to help those build their health and happiness for lifelong satisfaction. To this end, I have recommended below the four things we can all learn to grow and sustain long-term relationships. Turn LEFT will help your connections from the very start.

The L of LEFT stands for Listen. Good relationships start with acceptance of the other as they are and constructive listening will win you more friends than any other social skill. To listen with genuine interest can be developed with practice. Consider looking them in the eye whilst they are speaking. Also, you must avoid interrupting while they are talking. When someone keeps speaking without a break, it can be due to anxiety or the lack of listening support afforded them in childhood. Constructive listening will often break this cycle.

Consider the most asked question when two people who are already acquainted meet up. "How are you?" Most people have no interest in how they are as they never listen to the answer. It is better to ask a more specific question, like how is your back? How is your son getting on at school? Etc.

The E of LEFT is concerned with Encouragement. Society is the poorer for a lack of encouragement. Building long-tern relationships is rooted in encouraging others in their endeavours in all experiences of life. Regular encouragement does not need to be sycophantic or flattering. There is always something good to be found in any situation and we aim to identify and isolate the good element and encourage it.

The F of LEFT is Forgiveness. Practise forgiveness in the little things. When someone has been truly forgiven for a small indiscretion, they will value you and want to commit. Of course, there are exceptions but that doesn't matter as we all aim to develop mutually beneficial relationships. Those who refuse to connect are not worth concern. Focus on those who do.

The T of LEFT stands for Trust. To gain someone's trust, we need to always follow through with promises. Our word is our bond as reliability is a highly-sought after asset in someone and somewhat rare in modern society. Try not to agree to do things unless you are confident you can execute the commitment. In the long term, you win more respect and trust.

An example of real trust occurs in this short anecdote. An employer asked her secretary when answering the phone to tell the caller that she was in a meeting and could not speak. This was a lie as the boss was sitting at her desk with little to do. The secretary replied, "I am not going to lie for you." The employer then rebuked the secretary for disobedience to which the secretary responded, "If I can lie for you, I can lie to you when it is to my advantage." A mature employer will pick this up and can trust this secretary in bigger matters.

Trust is built over time. Trust within the world of personal as well as commercial relationships grows through the application of the four elements of LEFT. At the beginning of the chapter, I stated to turn LEFT. As a final thought, once you have built a friendship, keep going straight. To continue to turn left will eventually bring you back to where you started. In other words, be consistent with your behaviour and you will acquire life-long and deep connections.

WATER

We are made up of about 70% water and as such it is very important to keep hydrated. Most people will get by with two to three litres a day in cool climates but if you are in high temperatures or are physically active, then you might need considerably more. The symptoms of dehydration include headaches and in the case of extremely hot environments, heat exhaustion or even sunstroke. As your urine flow becomes less regular and much stronger with a deep yellow or even an orange tint, you are likely to be dehydrated.

When should you drink water? I think it is best to sip small amounts regularly throughout the day. Avoid taking a lot at night, otherwise, it will disturb your sleep by constantly having to visit the toilet in the small hours. Ordinary water is best because if it is in tea or coffee it will act as a diuretic which makes you urinate more often. The colour of your urine should be a pale yellow, a light straw colour.

In hot climates, water can often be contaminated with microbes of bacteria and viruses. Avoid foods that have been washed in local water and drink bottled water. If you are travelling to these countries from a temperate climate take precautions when drinking the water. It should be boiled before drinking. It can also be filtered and sterilised with a tablet to kill any pathogens that might cause sickness. Ultraviolet light also has some sterilising effects. Indigenous peoples of hotter climates are often immune to these pathogens and these days sterilisation plants are appearing in many of the larger, more developed cities.

When fasting, keep up your water intake and between meals, water should be taken as it is required for heathy digestion. Finally, rehydration following waterborne sicknesses should contain a tablespoon of sugar and a pinch of salt per litre. You can get rehydration salts to help with rehydration. Water can also be an aid to weight loss and makes you feel fuller after eating.

SUNLIGHT

In recent times sunlight has got a bad rap. The concern aroused from overexposure to the sun and the associated Melanoma has put people off enjoying the sun altogether. Some sunlight is good for you and will stimulate the production of vitamin D which helps build your immunity to many medical conditions and diseases. It is bad to get sunburnt and any prolonged exposure should include a high factor sun barrier cream. Any newly-appearing moles or skin lesions that get bigger or change colour, should be examined by a medical professional as skin cancer is usually treatable if caught early.

However, exposing yourself to some UV light from the sun for about twenty minutes a day has a net beneficial effect. A moderate amount of sun on your skin will also help with your mood and act as a positive support for depressive illness. Try spending some time in the early morning sun. It is good for your body to face it but never look at the sun and wear good-quality sunglasses.

CONTAGIOUS DISCIPLINE

Developing self-discipline is probably the most important single way to obtain optimum health and happiness. The interesting thing about self-discipline is that it is contagious to both you and others. Those who are consistently disciplined in one area find it easier to be disciplined in others. Also, the positive effects are seen in others because it encourages them to do the same.

Someone who is disciplined about their diet is more likely to exercise, be less wasteful with money and probably have better relationships all round. Self-discipline starts as capital where we only have so much to use up. After a time, it becomes income where we generate more discipline as we go along.

Start with something very small. Get up earlier in the morning by say 10 minutes. Do a short, unpleasant task before you take on other more attractive ventures. If possible, delay a meal by ten minutes from yesterday. The more you discipline yourself in the small things, the more it will grow. It is like compound interest; it accrues over time.

Bill Gates of Microsoft fame said that we overestimate what we can do in one week but underestimate what we can achieve in ten years. Many books have been written about how a slight change in habitual behaviour over time compounds to a very different life and it doesn't take all that long to develop good habits. A weight loss of 2 lbs weekly (roughly a kilogram) represents 100 lbs in one year, nearly 50 kilograms in just 12 months. All things are possible if you take it in small chunks over a sustained period.

STRESS CONTROL

There are three elements to the mental issues experienced by most people these days. Stress is wrongly associated with anxiety and worry. Stress is solely about how we are "wired up" to respond to danger, known as the three Fs. These animal responses to danger are Fight, Flight or Freeze and we are no different.

Anxiety, on the other hand, is depression projected into the future and is the way we emotionally react to stressful situations.

Worry is more to do with our rational analytical approach. In my experience, the cause of most bad habits like overeating is the result of anxiety. Stress causes people to avoid eating as they don't want to be digesting when running from that "tiger". We use worry as an insurance scheme to justify our anxiety, largely a feeling. Many people think "If I feel bad, I must have something to worry about."

Many of today's anxieties are related to media and digital input that continuously warns us of dangers all around. Fear is a great controller; it has been used by religions for thousands of years to get apathetic individuals to behave themselves. Today, the new religions, like the health police, continuously frighten people into believing the worst is about to happen. When you follow the guidelines in this book, you can relax. You are doing everything you can to keep yourself healthy, have good relationships and live a balanced life.

There are many interventions available to support you if you have excess stress. Coping with life's difficulties is more than practising a series of techniques, rather it concerns an attitude of mind and this is what I would like to address in this chapter.

The fundamental issue is a fear of uncertainty. People cannot cope with the uncertainty of life and with constant media input this uncertainty is magnified. If you are struggling with bills, health, family etc. you are experiencing suffering. The anxiety, however, is not so much the struggle, but uncertainty concerning the future that makes the struggle so mentally taxing.

Life by its very nature is uncertain and I believe we need to embrace this when exposed to mental illness. I have a history of anxiety, depression and dread about the future. However, I have found by taking action in the areas I can, i.e. what is mentioned in this book, I have managed to accept those things that I cannot change in the future by doing my best in the present.

That aside, the following things will help you with anxiety: therapy and counselling; mindfulness; exercise in all its forms; socialising with friends and relatives (the ones you get on with); forgiveness; avoiding stimulants in diet; sleep; taking action to deal with specific problems and avoiding procrastination; laughter; hobbies and distracting interests; prescribed medication if required; complementary treatments as mentioned in the relevant chapter and breathing techniques. As you can see these are all things discussed in this book and if you follow just 10% of the advice, your stress will come under control.

ABUSE

I think this is worth mentioning here as it is damaging to optimum health. Most people are not abusive but a significant minority will come into this category. There are many forms of abuse with three standing out as the most common and destructive to society. They are sexual abuse, physical abuse and psychological abuse. Some abusers combine all three, using one to leverage the other two. Within the area of sexual abuse, there is a prevalence of women being abused by partners, relatives, acquaintances and strangers. Most sexual abuse, however, is carried out in a domestic setting by close partners and relatives of the abuser.

Fortunately, this whole area has become more talked about in recent times and exposure is the single biggest factor in reducing the cases. Most abusers continue because they think they won't get caught. Where minors are involved, the law is tightening up on abuse but with adults, there is still an abusive epidemic in society.

Physical abuse takes place between children as well as adults and is often easier to detect than sexual abuse as it can involve physical damage to the body. This can occur between the same gender as well as between male and female.

The final type of abuse is one of the most difficult to detect and handle, psychological abuse. This can occur in the workplace, institutions and domestic environments. Abusers of all forms were often abused themselves when younger, often in childhood.

In essence, abuse is about power and control. It is seen in the animal kingdom where the alpha male will abuse weaker members of the tribe to secure the favours of the females. You could say this is natural but humans take it to a whole new level. In summary, people abuse simply because they can and intend to get away with it.

I have a few recommendations for those abused and those who might be in the future. Firstly, tell someone. The shame preventing victims from admitting abuse will only cause it to continue. Find a confidante you can go to and who will take the relevant action as soon as you are ready to expose the abuser. With psychological abuse, I would recommend courses in assertiveness. The power of the tongue to stop abusers in their tracks can be learned in these courses. Physical abuse rarely takes place if the individual is not frightened of the potential abuser. To this end, consider training in the martial arts or self-defence. It cannot guarantee freedom from abuse but it gives the potential victim confidence which will put the abuser off. Ninety-nine per cent of abusers are bullies and cowards and will soon capitulate when challenged.

AVOIDING COGNITIVE DECLINE (DEMENTIA)

As we age, our general cognitive function seems to diminish which is often associated with dementia. Much of what is defined as dementia is not a malfunction but the result of attitude and lifestyle.

This chapter is all about how you can minimise the effects of age-related cognitive performance, and improve your memory and general analytical and rational thinking.

1 Sleep

Make sure you are getting enough sleep. I have already mentioned sleep in a previous chapter and reiterate it here. The main reason that older people often drift off to sleep during the day is a way of protecting their brains from damage.

2 Stimulate the mind in several areas

The brain will build more neurological pathways through multiple rather than single stimuli. Do as many of these as you can. You don't have to be very good at them, you just need to work on improving your performance. Learn a new language, learn to play an instrument, do IQ and puzzle problems, crosswords, chess, read, write creatively, watch YouTube videos on educational subjects, converse, teach, learn memory techniques and study any subject in detail.

3 Exercise every day

I recommend about 30 minutes to include 20 minutes of (raised heart rate) aerobic activity.

4 Socialise

Mixing with other people helps the brain to function well and reduces depression and anxiety. Activities that combine exercise with socialising like dancing are especially useful.

5 Diet

Diet affects both brain protein and vascular decline so it is important to eat the correct food as mentioned earlier in this book. Fish oils and nuts should be a part of your diet. Avoid alcohol and smoking as much as possible and drink plenty of water.

6 Find a reason to get up in the morning

Caring for loved ones and friends and the community at large is excellent. If you don't know what you are going to do today, you must try and find something. If you like your work, only retire if you must and keep working as long as possible. No law in nature says you must retire at 65. Consider starting your own business even if you are in your sixties. It is never too late to start something new.

FINANCIAL SECURITY

It is a sad fact that wealthier people live longer, are more healthy and generally happier than the poor. I will break down the different income levels around the world to show why wealth is a good indicator of health.

The abject poor are at the bottom of the financial ladder and do not have enough to eat. Being malnourished severely compromises their health, shortens life and gives them a poor lifestyle. They usually have no access to gainful employment and spend their whole lives trying to get food for themselves and their families. They also live in areas prone to conflict and natural disasters.

The next group is the **financially surviving.** This community conversely has far too much work and is having to slog for 18 hours a day just to eat. They have no time to learn about money and have no access to higher education where most of the world's wealth is located. They live longer than the previous group and secure survival through having large families.

The next group is the **financially adequate.** They have access to health care and education but have to pay for it at the point of need. They are subject to tax and unlikely to have enough time to focus on their health. They provide most of the manual and manufacturing labour in the world. Their families are smaller and they have aspirations for their children to succeed through business and professional careers. This group often have a better chance of emigrating and makes up a high percentage of the world's refugees. They search for an economy that is more affluent and secure.

The following community is the **financially secure** These are people with excess money. They can choose where to live and select better areas for air quality etc. Their education has alerted them to the risks of a poor lifestyle and are most concerned about the environment. Having received an education they focus on their health and that of their children. They have a stake in the community such as owning property and land and ensure their children have good health and education.

The final group is the **financially abundant,** the superrich. They have lots of investments, cash and access to more money. This group does not live as well as the financially secure as they fall prey to the temptations of excess wealth, including narcotics and weight gain. They often feel that they can live an extravagant life as their money will protect them from the consequences of a poor lifestyle.

If you are reading this book, you are possibly in the middle section, between the financially surviving and the financially secure. Those at either end of the spectrum feel they would have no interest in this book.

You must understand that your wealth directly affects your health and lifespan. It also increases the health of the generations to come. On this point, you owe it to yourself to get educated about money. Accounting, budgeting, investing, compounding, and the difference between assets and liabilities. Learn as much as you can about financial numeracy, financial literacy and business trends in financial journalism. Your job might have nothing to do with money so you must study it as a separate life-saving subject. Use social media, go on courses and start to practise the skills obtained to raise your standard of living and subsequent health.

GETTING CHECKED OUT

Many conditions threaten our health, especially as we age. If we live in a developed society, there are plenty of opportunities to avoid or at least lessen the effects of these conditions by getting regular checks before symptoms occur.

1 Cardio Vascular diseases

This is common to both sexes and is largely a result of lifestyle but can be genetic as well. The areas for checks are cholesterol level, blood pressure and the conditions of the arterial and vascular blood vessels around the heart, organs and brain.

Regular checkups through blood tests etc. are essential to reveal potential risks. Treatment would include blood pressure, anti-coagulant and statin medication. Also, lifestyle changes, including dietary changes, more exercise, more sleep and stress management all play their part. The biggest causes of cardiovascular diseases are neglecting checkups, not taking medication and an unwillingness to change lifestyle accordingly. Lung conditions can also be alleviated if periodically checked out by a chest doctor.

Total blood screening should be carried out once a year from fifty years plus to check that the organs are functioning well as with blood sugar.

2 Cancer

There are many types of cancer and again most can be avoided or minimised by having regular checks and taking appropriate action early. Prostate cancer kills men because they don't get checked out. The prostate specific antigen (PSA) can indicate an enlarged prostate which might be benign but a blood test biopsy and an MRI scan will confirm this. If cancer is found early, effective treatment is very likely.

With women, a smear test is essential to check for cervical cancer and the regular feeling examination of their breasts to find lumps would also be beneficial. Men should also check their testicles for abnormal lumps every couple of months.

If either sex discovers symptoms that are different from the usual, visit the doctor. Many communities are introducing national screening which helps detect possible conditions. Bowel screenings on a two-yearly basis are becoming common where excrement can be checked for occult blood, a sign of bowel cancer whilst individuals are encouraged to look for changes in bowel habits, pain and overt dark blood in stools.

3 Senses

Regular eye and ear tests at two-year intervals should occur in those over forty and younger if there is a history of sensory problems. It is also necessary to have regular dental checks as a buildup of bacteria from untreated mouth and gum infections can be detrimental to general health.

4 Feet

This might seem trivial compared with some of the topics we have been talking about, but feet are very important. If your feet are giving you trouble, you will be less able to exercise and that will have a detrimental effect on your general health. Get them treated by a chiropodist as soon as they present problems so you can keep mobile.

5 Lungs

The best way we can clean our lungs is to spend as much time surrounded by nature and to stop smoking. Smoking kills millions of people a year and is the product of cravings and habits. The cravings are the result of a physical addiction and the habit is the result of emotional addiction. It is almost impossible to break the physical craving until you break the emotional habits that underlie your behaviour. If you imagine that a craving is the effect of the accelerator in your car, then the habit is the effect of the gear.

You can't drive at 70 miles an hour in first gear and that is what people try to do by attempting to stop smoking without changing their habits. I do not want to make this book about smoking as I can't do it justice here but if you email me at my address mentioned earlier in this book, I can give you some advice on how to break a habit chain.

6 Diabetes

This is one of the most endemic conditions in the developed world and is increasing in underdeveloped communities year by year. There are two major types of diabetes, Type One and Type

Two. Type One can be genetic and might be triggered by a shock or other medical conditions. Type Two is generally age-related and mainly the result of lifestyle.

The good news concerning Type Two is that it is largely avoidable and can in certain incidences, be reversed if the correct lifestyle changes are implemented. As with most other conditions, diet plays its part which should consist of low sugar and carbohydrates. This will help to reduce another factor and that is obesity and Body Mass Index (BMI). Reducing alcohol consumption and preferably cutting it out would be ideal, whilst smoking should be avoided. I recommend that plenty of exercise will also help to alleviate the symptoms as aerobic exercise uses up sugar. Again, regular checks of your blood sugar will indicate where your glycemic levels are and if diagnosis is confirmed, then this becomes a necessity. Insulin-dependent diabetics are usually committed to medication for life but those who are pre-diabetic can reverse the condition.

I recommend that you take your blood sugar seriously from an early age as sustained hyperglycaemia leads to many other conditions as we age. Lethargy and a constant desire to urinate could suggest you might be pre-diabetic.

Many other conditions need checks, like the risk of aortic aneurysms, but this is a one-off check and if found negative would not need repeating. The main point of this chapter is to emphasise that any checks offered or that you can afford should be done regularly to reduce the risk of chronic or acute illness in an ageing population.

PATHOGENIC DISEASE

In the developing world, two disease types kill millions of people every year. The poor in the third world don't develop cancer and heart disease so much as they die from pathogens before these mature conditions become apparent.

They are bacterial and viral diseases. Bacteria are the most successful living organisms on the planet and are believed to have existed on Earth a billion years before any other living thing. These pathogens are treatable with antibiotics but are becoming resistant to many of the current crops of antibiotic medication in the Western world. Conditions like c difficile and MRSA are a big problem, especially in hospitals where the patient's health is already compromised. The problem is the overuse of antibiotics causing bacteria to mutate to survive. We all need to use fewer antibiotics and fight off many common ailments where the lack of medication is not a major health risk.

The second group of pathogens are viruses which are not living entities and will only replicate within host cells. The planet has just experienced this phenomenon through the COVID-19 epidemic. General hygiene is essential to protect us as the immune system functions very well in healthy bodies.

I think, however, that excessive sterilisation of everything is not good as it does not allow the body to build up resistance to many common conditions. The immune system needs something to fight and the mixing of children at school and play builds a stronger genetic pool for future generations. Serious conditions need to be vaccinated against but many common ailments should be allowed to take their course.

Finally, there are several ways that pathogens can enter the body, via water, food, air and through physical contact. When we refer to contagious diseases, we think of conditions like hepatitis B and HIV. Influenza is airborne and cholera is waterborne. Global travel has caused these diseases to spread so all the normal precautions should be applied. Wash your hands before eating; sterilise or boil water before drinking; avoid foods that are not properly cooked and make sure you are fully inoculated against any disease prevalent in the places you are visiting.

OPTIMUM HEALTH THROUGH A COMPLEMENTARY APPROACH

First, I would like to explain that I believe complementary medicine is just that, not an alternative. Some complementary treatments are much older than conventional Western medicine and have their place in good health.

The fundamental difference between the two is one of approach. Complementary medicine is often designed as preventative, a prophylactic preventing health breakdown in the first place. In ancient China, doctors were paid when their clients were well and only stopped getting paid when their patients became ill. Modern medicine is based on how to treat existing conditions, though this is beginning to change.

Many people feel that treatments like homoeopathy are highly effective, whereas others believe it is total quackery. I knew a homoeopath and was at that time very sceptical. The fee he charged seemed high until I discovered he was also a conventional consultant physician who could charge five times the amount for a consultation in traditional medicine.

I am totally in favour of medicine that has been proven scientifically through double-blind trials and experimentation within medical facilities and hospitals. However, I do not think one needs to exclude the other. The argument that wellness is simply a result of the placebo effect (getting well because you think the treatment is effective) is not the whole story. Traditional medicine also uses it.

A client of mine described how her husband couldn't sleep. He was taking some strong sleeping pills which greatly concerned my client. She approached her General Practitioner and asked for advice. Her doctor conspired with her to reduce the strength of the sleeping pill over a period without telling the husband what was going on. He continued to have good sleep until there was no active ingredient in the medication at all. The classically trained doctor used the placebo effect within his own discipline.

We all have a natural ability to heal, given half a chance and many conditions will cure themselves in time, using the immune system within the body. That said, never underestimate the mind as a tool for improving general health. We know little about how the mind works and in time, we could discover it plays a much bigger part in general wellness than is currently perceived.

The golden rule is this: prevent what you can through a wide range of health interventions and subsequently treat conditions that present themselves, firstly by conventional medicine and secondly through a complementary approach. Be careful of contraindications; that is one treatment or prophylactic might interfere with another. Reading labels and getting professional advice will ensure a safe approach to this issue.

Here are 12 of the main, established, qualification-based complementary therapists who treat a wide range of conditions across the world.

1 Homeopaths

The theory that like-treats-like, Homeopathy is based on adding water to an active ingredient to produce a highly diluted form. It is based on the concept of water having a "memory" and the diluted form is more effective than the undiluted version.

2 Herbal Treatments Therapists

The irony of this approach is that often the active ingredient taken from plants is similar to that provided in classical medicine hidden in a pill. This isn't always the case but biochemical interventions are often judged by the way they are offered, not what is offered. It has its base in ancient Chinese medicine.

3 Acupuncturists

This stimulates the central nervous system by using needles to release curative chemicals in the muscles, spine and brain.

4 Alexander Technique therapists

This is based on how changes in posture and movement can treat acquired bad habits.

5 Aromatherapists

Aromatherapy uses essential oils in various forms, including inhaling and massage to treat many conditions including stress.

6 Chiropractic therapists

These therapists use pressure to manipulate joints and to correct misalignments with the spine.

7 Osteopaths

Massage and manipulate the skeleton tissue and muscle etc. They differ from Chiropractors in that they focus on the whole body.

8 Hypnotherapists

Hypnosis is a therapy that uses an induced level of trance or heightened suggestion to guide a client to favourable outcomes, using the resources of their unconscious mind.

9 Reflexologists

This is used to treat stress and conditions by manipulating and massaging the feet. The meridians of reflexology can also be found in the hands and head.

10 Naturopaths

This technique provides treatment for certain conditions without advocating the requirement for traditional drugs. It focuses on diet and exercise as a recommended approach.

11 Counsellors

Counselling is a listening therapy that guides the client to solve their own problems through using highly creative listening.

12 Psychotherapists

Psychotherapy is more of a talking therapy with many different models of psychological intervention. It usually requires clients to carry out therapeutic homework between sessions.

EMERGENCY

This chapter is more about protecting the health and lives of your loved ones, friends and acquaintances. It is in no way designed to replace a first aid course which I would recommend everyone takes from a recognised provider. If you do not know how to go about this, get in touch with me via email and I can advise you accordingly.

Having said all that, I would like to cover some of the basic issues concerned with emergency conditions to guide you to provide optimum health and safety for your family.

I will start with a few definitions. A diagnosis is arrived at from the combination of history, signs and symptoms. Triage is about prioritising conditions according to their seriousness. The primary assessment is concerned with airways, breathing and circulation of the blood. The secondary survey is concerned with other conditions that might compromise life if left unchecked. Trauma is what occurs to a casualty externally and medical is generated and caused internally. A heart attack would be classed as medical and a road traffic incident would be classed as trauma.

EMERGENCY - THE PRIMARY SURVEY

DR HELP ABC

This is the primary survey in practice. The D stands for Danger where the first aid provider needs to ensure their own safety before attending to the casualty's needs. Examples of danger are fire, gas, water/river/sea, electricity, aggressive casualties and/or bystanders, broken glass, falling masonry, chemicals etc. If any of these dangers exist, be cautious. You might need to get professional help before proceeding any further.

The R of DR stands for Response. Within the non-hospital/paramedic community there are only four levels of response. They are summarised in the word AVPU. This stands for Aware, Responding to Voice, responding to Pain and Unresponsive.

You would notice if a casualty is responsive and if not, you should ask them questions. If they don't respond to questions, then flick their ear or nose with a small sensation of pain. If this doesn't work, they can be said to be unresponsive and unconscious.

If the casualty is unconscious, you will need to get help, both professionally and from those around you. Use your mobile to call the emergency services (numbers vary around the world) UK is 112/999, US is 911 etc. Give the telephone responder information as to where the incident is and any further comments on what happened (history).

It is now time to check the A of the ABC which stands for Airways. This is done by checking that the airways are clear and a tilting back of the head. (Only practise this in a supervised first aid course.)

Once a clear airway is established, check the B of ABC, Breathing. This is done by placing your ear close to the casualty's mouth and listening for breathing. It is also helpful if you place the **back of your hand** (for modesty with female casualties) on the casualty's chest to feel for respiratory movement.

If the casualty is breathing whilst being unconscious, carry out a quick sweep to see if there are any other injuries, especially spinal damage, and place them in the recovery position. This position has the casualty turned on their front with one leg drawn up and the back of one of their hands resting under the face. Practise this process on a recognised and supervised first aid course.

If the casualty is not breathing, you will need to apply Cardio-Pulmonary Resuscitation (CPR). This involves compressing the chest just above the sternum thirty times as demonstrated by your first aid trainer. Expired Air Respiration (EAR) has also been used between periods of CPR. This involves blowing your exhaled breath twice into the casualty's lungs by sealing their mouth around yours and squeezing their nose. The risk of infection has made this a less popular option these days which can be overcome with one-way breathing filter masks, airbags and the like. If you can't bring yourself to carry out EAR at least do the CPR.

Note, these days if the casualty is not breathing, assume there is no circulation but this can be checked by feeling the pulse (pressed where an artery goes over a bone). Dilated pupils and bluish lips are also signs. The carotid artery is a good place to locate the pulse. It is found by placing two fingers beside the windpipe of the throat, about halfway up the neck.

EMERGENCY - CAUSES OF UNCONSCIOUSNESS

FISH SHAPED

The F of FISH stands for Fainting

Definition: a temporary loss of oxygen to the brain.

Causes: fatigue, infection, malnutrition, psychological shock etc.

Signs and symptoms: temporary unconsciousness, pale face (ashen grey), pale lips, collapse.

Treatment: lie casualty down, reassure, raise legs, and treat cause if appropriate.

I of FISH stands for Internal injuries

Definition: mainly damage to blood vessels from fractures etc.

Causes: various types of trauma, and some medical conditions like aneurysms and haemorrhage.

Signs and Symptoms: shock, pale face that does not respond well to treatment. Compromised breathing and circulation etc.

Treatment: Get emergency help as soon as possible; monitor their airways and breathing, even when in the recovery position. If necessary, carry out CPR. and EAR.

The S of FISH stands for Shock

Definition: a lack of circulating oxygenated blood to the vital organs.

Causes: bleeding, psychological, extremes of temperature, burns, electricity, infections, heart conditions etc.

Signs and symptoms: pale face/lips, a rapid, shallow heartbeat, rapid shallow breathing (hyperventilation).

Treatment: Treat the cause, get help, lie the casualty down, raise legs, reassure even if unconscious and keep warm (but not too hot) with plenty of air and rest.

H of FISH stands for Heart attack

Definition: the death of cells damaging the muscle of the heart.

Causes: genetic, lifestyle, including diet, lack of exercise, cholesterol, high blood pressure, clogged arteries etc.

Signs and symptoms: pale face, extreme pain in the chest and down the arm, terror if conscious and irregular heartbeat.

Note: A heart attack is not necessarily a cardiac arrest. The latter means that the heartbeat has ceased or has an irregular rhythm and can be the result of many conditions other than a heart attack.

Treatment: Sit down with the knees raised, and legs in 'W' position. Reassure and carry out the procedures of the primary survey above if unconscious. Support with medication only if the person is known to you; the medication has been prescribed for this condition to this individual; you are fully conversant with their condition and a doctor has approved your assistance.

The S of SHAPED stands for a Stroke

Definition: A stroke is the result of a lack of blood to the brain due to a blockage or a bleed and renders the casualty partially paralysed.

Causes: lifestyle, associated with high blood pressure, genetic propensity.

Signs and symptoms: red face, drooping mouth, paralysis usually down one side, distress, sometimes problems with verbal communication, possible unconsciousness.

Treatment: Call an ambulance ASAP, sit up, reassure, support the paralysed side, and monitor for primary survey DR Help ABC.

The H of SHAPED stands for Head injury

Definition: varies due to trauma.

Causes: as above.

Signs and symptoms: headache, pupils not reacting to light, poor reflexes, possible concussion/compression.

Treatment: Get help. Assume potential concussion (the shaking of the brain against the skull) monitor for DR Help ABC. Compression is a possible result of concussion where a bleed in the brain can clot and press on the brain tissue which can be fatal. An operation is required ASAP.

The A of SHAPED stands for Asphyxia

Definition: insufficient oxygen arriving to the lungs for adequate respiration.

Causes: choking, swelling of airways through poison or allergic reaction, mouth and/or nose being covered or badly damaged due to trauma, anaphylaxis, strangulation.

Signs and symptoms: distress, red face, inability to produce a productive cough, leading to unconsciousness.

Treatment: Ambulance! Attempt to remove any foreign object from the mouth. Give Epipen if anaphylaxis is the cause and you are trained to use one. Use backslaps or the Hymnic Manoeuvre to clear airways. (To be practised on the first aid course.) DR Help ABC if unconscious

The P of SHAPED stands for Poison

Definition: two types: narcotic and non-narcotic. Narcotic poisons can be safe to take if prescribed in the right doses but will become toxic if overdosed. We could include alcohol in this example. Non-narcotic poisons are those that are toxic even in small amounts.

Causes: inhaled, ingested, injected, absorbed.

Signs and symptoms: numerous.

Treatment: If possible, establish which poison has been taken. Has it been inhaled, absorbed, injected or ingested? DR Help ABC. Keep casualty conscious if possible. Be careful the poison does not affect you.

The E of SHAPED stands for Epilepsy

Definition: an electrochemical distortion of the brain.

Causes: can be generic or might be the result of trauma, especially head injuries.

Signs and symptoms: Petit Mal - casualty seems vague and disturbed, won't necessarily lose consciousness. Grand Mal - includes muscle tightening, muscle spasms, pale face, collapse and distress. Note: Status epilepticus is a continuous state of having seizures. The casualty must attend hospital as soon as possible.

Treatment: Avoid close contact with the casualty but try to protect them when collapse occurs. Make sure the head does not bang on anything. Once the spasms are over, place them in the recovery position. Check vital signs for airway, breathing etc. as before.

The D of SHAPED - Diabetes

This condition has already been covered in this book. There are two ways a diabetic might react. These are hypoglycaemia and hyperglycaemia. Po rhymes with low and low blood sugar is more serious in the short term than high blood sugar. If you think the casualty might be diabetic, give them something sweet ASAP. This will protect them from the risks of too much insulin and if they already have too much sugar then a little more won't be bad in the immediate term. If they don't recover, assume hyperglycaemia. Get medical help and support diabetic medication if appropriate.

ADDITIONS TO EMERGENCY PROTOCOLS

Positioning of casualty

Before moving anyone, bear in mind there might be spinal damage and movement should only occur if absolutely necessary.

1 If the face is pale, raise the tail (legs) raised lying down.

2 If the face is red, raise the head, and sit up.

3 If the face is blue, the extremities of lips, nose etc. it is over to you. That means you need to carry out a Primary Survey (DR HELP ABC).

External Bleeding

Arterial bleeds are from vessels leaving the heart, are bright red and in every case but one, contain oxygen. The bleed occurs with the rhythm of the heartbeat. Venial bleeds are steady and produce darker, deoxygenated blood. Capillary bleeds from small vessels trickle and are rarely serious.

The four ways to stop external bleeds.

Direct pressure:

1 Direct pressure on the wound with your gloved hands. Using bandages etc. is also helpful for direct pressure.

2 Application of up to three bandages on top of wound and secured with a knot or safety pin.

Indirect pressure:

3 Pressure points. This involves pressing on an arterial junction above a limb to stop blood from entering the limb.

4 Tourniquets. Tying knotted material tightly over joints to stop bleeding from entering the limb.

Note: First Aiders are not encouraged to apply pressure points or tourniquets as these are only used when moving a casualty and are in the realm of the professional. A tourniquet that is not released every few minutes can cause gangrene. A First Aider aims to keep the casualty still and get professionals to come to them.

Protocol with water rescue

If someone is in water, (the worst environment for causing hypothermia), follow this protocol to get them out.

1 Reach

2 Throw

3 Wade

4 Row

5 Tow with a towing aid

6 Tow

In other words, don't enter the water unless it is safe to do so and only make contact with the casualty as a last resort. In the UK, the Royal Life Saving Society runs excellent courses on how to rescue in water. I recommend you contact them for available dates. Note, you need to be able to swim to take these courses. If you don't swim, consider learning; it could save your life. The cycling proficiency test is another one to consider if you are cycling on busy roads.

Fire

The triangle of fire says that fire requires three items to burn: oxygen, fuel and heat. If you remove one of these, the fire will subside and eventually go out. If the fire is electrical, use a CO_2 extinguisher rather than a water one and call the fire service if it is beyond your control. Do not put water on fires that are the result of oils, as in kitchens. Cover with a fire blanket, available from most general stores.

PRIORITISING SURVIVAL AND OPTIMUM HEALTH IN CONFLICT AND WILDERNESS SITUATIONS

When exposed to an environment that is threatening to life and general health, there is a set of timed priorities that you need to consider when preparing to survive. They are timed as they are in descending order of importance. In the modern business environment, it is suggested that you should attempt to do what is important above what is urgent. In the game of survival, the opposite is true. The most urgent must be completed first.

1 Physical danger from aggressive personnel and animals

The most dangerous situations are where there is conflict or where wild animals might attack causing immediate fatality. It is important to understand that small poisonous creatures kill more people than the larger animals. Most of nature is frightened of humanity but those that are strong enough will fight rather than run away. The hippopotamus is probably the most dangerous large animal to people, followed by the big cats, elephants and the like. Smaller animals, snakes, spiders and jellyfish can contain some of the most toxic venom.

When it comes to human conflict, alien individuals and travellers are at risk from stray ballistics, kidnapping for ransom and summary execution on suspicion of spying.

When visiting any country do your research and follow government guidelines about the potential conflict risks. Governmental and non-governmental organisations operating in conflict situations have local counterparts; they will smooth the way to providing emergency relief operations which are often backed by armed military, such as United Nations Peacekeeping troops. Local knowledge is everything so make sure you have good backup and support before you venture into unstable countries.

2 Fire

I would put fire above water as the next most urgent consideration. Others may disagree, but Hypothermia can kill quicker than dehydration and the requirement to boil water to make it safe to drink is not possible without fire. Animals of all sizes are frightened of fire and being close to a fire can deter an attack.

Starting a fire can be difficult but you will need fuel, usually wood in the wilderness. You will also need some way of creating a spark like matches or a flint stone. When starting the fire, the wood will need to be dry so collecting kindling and keeping it in a pocket or under your shirt might be the only option when it is raining. Fires are built up from small kindling twigs to larger and larger timbers culminating in extensive logs. Fires will need to be fanned to help further ignition. This can be done with any flat-ish surface acting as a sail beside the fire. Blowing into the fire can also create vigorous burning. Further logs are stored near the fire to dry them out before burning. You will need to continue collecting wood to keep the fire going. If you want to know more about this or any other survival technique, I recommend John (Lofty) Wiseman's book, SAS Survival Handbook which is very comprehensive.

3 Water

When camping out you need to locate close to the water source, as your energy will quickly deteriorate due to lack of nutrition and you don't want to have to go walking miles to find water. Fast-flowing rivers are the best as any dead animals upstream will have their toxic pathogens washed downstream before you drink from the river. Your fire will allow you to ensure sterile water by boiling it for some minutes and allowing it to cool before it can be drunk.

Salt water should not be drunk so sea water is in effect poisonous as it upsets the osmotic salt balance in the system which quickly becomes fatal. In damp climates, it is possible to collect fresh water in containers, especially with the nightly dew.

I have heard the quote that you can live for three minutes without air, three days without water and three weeks without food. This is a huge generalisation. When in hot and humid environments or when suffering from an infection, you will start dehydrating very quickly so you will need to find a water source within a day. Eating food without water is also problematic as you need water to aid digestion and eating will make you crave water even more.

4 Food

I will again defer to John (Lofty) Wiseman's book about selecting edible food. He is an expert in this field and takes the topic much further than the scope of this book. He also includes the skills of hunting and trapping, as animal protein is highly nutritious in survival situations. The very carbohydrates and sugars that were rejected earlier in the book now come into their own as they will keep you alive for longer with the benefits of storing energy as fat.

5 Shelter

Once you have established a food supply, your next consideration is shelter. This will also help to protect you from the extreme cold, especially the ravages of wind and act as a shade in the extreme heat. Shelters rarely work first time if using natural flora and fauna when constructing the dwelling. They will need to be improved upon when rain exposes all the holes within the shelter.

6 Protocols for awareness of the hypothermic response

Four factors will induce hypothermia from the extreme cold: poor nutrition, cold air, wind and cold water. The quickest transfer of heat is in the water and survival will be shorter than on land. Vigorous exercise will help survival at a campsite but in water, it will have the opposite effect. The more you move in the water, the colder you become. It is better to stay still.

On dry land, the next risk factor is wind as this takes heat from the body very quickly and it is here that a well-constructed shelter, out of the wind, could be a lifesaver.

Cold air temperature is less of a problem but can still induce hypothermia if the core body temperature drops a couple of degrees Celsius.

7 Sickness

Bacterial and Viral sickness is attracted to the malnourished and stressed victim of the elements and needs to be avoided as much as possible. These pathogens will enter the body through inhalation, ingestion and physical contact.

Avoid leaving food around as it can attract contaminated creatures. Contagious diseases are less common, provided you do not have physical contact with animals unless they are cooked. Avoid sexual contact in alien environments with those you do not know and avoid the sharing of body fluids. Fresh air is the best protection from picking up contaminants. Avoid insect bites by covering your skin from top to toe with clothing, especially between your ankles and your trousers. Mosquitos tend to bite at dawn and dusk when they prefer to feed. Keep your campsite away from swampy areas and not too close to the water supply.

8 Psychological Considerations

You will survive longer from the stress element than the previous seven topics but there is a risk that stress will undermine your resolve to apply the above. Survival is eighty per cent attitude and therefore stress is a consideration. Your focus, once you have secured the seven elements already mentioned, is to extract yourself from the situation and all your spare energy should be focused on how to get out. There are two famous examples of how stress was managed by focusing on escape from a hostile environment. One comes from fiction the other from war.

The first example is taken from the book 'Lord of the Flies' by the Nobel Laureate, William Golding. The hero of the story, about a group of children stranded on a desert island, was Ralph who tried to keep a fire going to alert a passing aircraft of their plight. He used the goal to get home as a way of keeping his sanity. Many of the other children turned into savages where survival was purely a matter of killing.

The other example is that of Colditz Castle, the German Prisoner of War camp. Many of the prisoners who were prominent PoWs from all branches of the Allied military spent all their spare time planning and attempting to escape. This focus kept them sane until their final liberation in 1945.

CONCLUSION

This book has covered a range of well-being approaches that I feel will put you on the path to a more fulfilled and contented life. The theme of the book is that of a holistic approach. One thing helps another. Exercise helps stress, sleep helps to avoid dementia which is also helped by exercise. A good diet helps us to exercise and helps with energy which helps with raising our income.

The world of experts is concentrating on a single issue for improved health which, when done in isolation, will not change lives significantly. People are jumping from one thing to another and finding few long-term solutions to their problems. The answer is to take small steps in all the areas discussed above. Don't overwhelm yourself with big steps in one discipline, such as changing your diet, as optimum health is the result of concurrent rather than consecutive action.

Peter Bull

FEEDBACK

I'd be delighted if you would take a minute and leave a review of this of any of my **GET IN TOUCH** books on *Amazon*, *Goodreads, Google* or other review site.

Thank you.

Peter Bull

ALSO IN THE GET IN TOUCH SERIES

I have found that succinct information that gets to the roots of what we seek to learn is highly effective. The **GET IN TOUCH** series of books and audiobooks is therefore designed to be short and to the point. Your feedback as a reader is always welcome, and more information on the GET IN TOUCH series can be found on my website:

www.getintouchbooks.com

GET IN TOUCH: With Your Public Voice

GET IT TOUCH: With Your Inner Wealth

GET IN TOUCH: With Your Slimmer Self

GET IN TOUCH: With Your Universe

GET IN TOUCH: With Your Better Mental Health

GET IN TOUCH: With Your Inner Genius

GET IN TOUCH: With Your Inner Quizmaster

GET IN TOUCH: With Your Startup Building Business

GET IN TOUCH: With Your Talking Heads

GET IN TOUCH: With Your Visual Thinking

GET IN TOUCH: With Your MAS Market

www.getintouchbooks.com

Direct: thebestsolution@icloud.com
Books: peter@getintouchbooks.com

linkedin.com/in/peterabull

Peter Bull Get in Touch Books

facebook.com/getintouchbooks

@getintouchbooks

Milton Keynes UK
Ingram Content Group UK Ltd.
UKHW020937201123
432908UK00022B/3285